Sukhbir Singh

Monograph On PRP In Hair Rejuvenation And Various Hair Disorders

Sukhbir Singh

Monograph On PRP In Hair Rejuvenation And Various Hair Disorders

Role Of PRP In Hair Disorders

LAP LAMBERT Academic Publishing

Impressum / Imprint
Bibliografische Information der Deutschen Nationalbibliothek: Die Deutsche Nationalbibliothek verzeichnet diese Publikation in der Deutschen Nationalbibliografie; detaillierte bibliografische Daten sind im Internet über http://dnb.d-nb.de abrufbar.
Alle in diesem Buch genannten Marken und Produktnamen unterliegen warenzeichen-, marken- oder patentrechtlichem Schutz bzw. sind Warenzeichen oder eingetragene Warenzeichen der jeweiligen Inhaber. Die Wiedergabe von Marken, Produktnamen, Gebrauchsnamen, Handelsnamen, Warenbezeichnungen u.s.w. in diesem Werk berechtigt auch ohne besondere Kennzeichnung nicht zu der Annahme, dass solche Namen im Sinne der Warenzeichen- und Markenschutzgesetzgebung als frei zu betrachten wären und daher von jedermann benutzt werden dürften.

Bibliographic information published by the Deutsche Nationalbibliothek: The Deutsche Nationalbibliothek lists this publication in the Deutsche Nationalbibliografie; detailed bibliographic data are available in the Internet at http://dnb.d-nb.de.
Any brand names and product names mentioned in this book are subject to trademark, brand or patent protection and are trademarks or registered trademarks of their respective holders. The use of brand names, product names, common names, trade names, product descriptions etc. even without a particular marking in this work is in no way to be construed to mean that such names may be regarded as unrestricted in respect of trademark and brand protection legislation and could thus be used by anyone.

Coverbild / Cover image: www.ingimage.com

Verlag / Publisher:
LAP LAMBERT Academic Publishing
ist ein Imprint der / is a trademark of
OmniScriptum GmbH & Co. KG
Heinrich-Böcking-Str. 6-8, 66121 Saarbrücken, Deutschland / Germany
Email: info@lap-publishing.com

Herstellung: siehe letzte Seite /
Printed at: see last page
ISBN: 978-3-659-64117-6

Copyright © 2014 OmniScriptum GmbH & Co. KG
Alle Rechte vorbehalten. / All rights reserved. Saarbrücken 2014

Monograph on PRP-Platelet Rich Plasma therapy in Hair Rejuvenation and various hair disorders

Author

Dr. Sukhbir Singh , M.S. Gen. Surgery, DNB Plastic surgery

Consultant Plastic and Cosmetic Surgeon (Ex Resident, Lok Nayak hospital)

Department of Burns, Plastic and aesthetic Surgery

Kamal Hospital, Kaushambhi, U.P., India

Name & address for correspondence:

Dr. Sukhbir singh   Consultant Plastic Surgeon

S-212, Greater kailash part 2,

New-Delhi-48, INDIA

Phone (r) 91-11-65194758

Mobile.91-9910391229

Email id: -sukhi21278@gmail.com,sukhi_1@yahoo.com

Table of Contents

S.No.		Page No.
1	Introduction	4-6
2	PRP-protocol for its preparation and its role in hair rejuvenation	7-20
3	PRP in Chronic Alopecia Areata- Our Centre Experience	21-33
4	Role of PRP in Primary Cicatricial Alopecia	34-44

Introduction

Platelet-rich plasma (PRP) is a platelet concentrate in a small plasma volume[1] which contains proteins such as fibrin, fibronectin and vitronectin. Several simplified protocols for the preparation of PRP have been developed to facilitate its clinical application.[2,3,4] According to Marx,[5] PRP should have a platelet concentration 300 to 400% greater than that of the whole blood in order to be considered a "therapeutic PRP." Both quantitative and qualitative analysis has to be done to ensure the best PRP for therapeutic efficacy. Various reagents have been used for harvesting of PRP. Similarly different centrifugation techniques (double and single) [6,7,8] have been compared for obtaining platelet concentrations. PRP presently is being used for several indications like musculoskeletal disorders, etc. apart from hair and facial rejuvenation.

The final sample obtained after ensuring a high platelet concentrate has to be used within 30 minutes of its preparation. It is injected in the scalp after local anaesthesia application in the subfollicular plane. Patients are sent home once the PRP session was over and they are in stable condition after checking all the vitals. They are called for review after 4 weeks for next session or earlier if any need arises.

References: -

1. Nagata H.J.M., et al. Effectiveness of two Methods for preparation of Autologous Platelet-Rich Plasma: An Experimental Study in Rabbits. Eur J Dent. 2010 October; 4(4): 395–402.

2. Anitua E. Plasma rich in growth factors: preliminary results of use in the preparation of sites for implants. Int J Oral Maxillofac Implants. 1999;14:529–53

3. Landesberg R, Roy M, Glickman RS. Quantification of growth factor levels using a simplified method of platelet-rich plasma gel preparation. J Oral Maxillofac Surg. 2000;58:297–300.

4. Sonnleitner D, Huemer P, Sullivan DY. A simplified technique for producing Platelet-rich plasma and Platelet Concentrate for intraoral bone grafting techniques: A technical note. Int J Oral Maxillofac Implants. 2000;15:879–882.

5. Marx RE. Platelet-rich plasma: evidence to support its use. J Oral Maxillofac Surg. 2004;62:489–496.

6. Marx RE, Carlson ER, Eichstaedt RM, Schimmele SR, Strauss JE, Georgeff KR. Platelet-rich plasma: Growth factor enhancement for bone grafts. Oral Surg Oral Med Oral Pathol Oral Radiol. 1998;85:638–646.

7. Anitua E. La utilización de los factores de crecimiento plasmáticos en cirugía oral, maxilofacial y periodoncia (PRGF) Rev Actual Odontoestomatol. 2001;6:305–315.

8. Eby EW. Platelet-rich plasma: Harvesting with a single-spin centrifuge. J Oral Implantol. 2002;28:297–301.

PRP-protocol for its preparation and its role in hair rejuvenation

Objectives

The purpose of this study was to study the protocol for preparation of platelet rich plasma (PRP) and to assess its effectiveness in hair rejuvenation.

Methods

The study was conducted at Kamal Hospital, Kaushambi. All the patients who had diffuse thinning of hairs, hair fall or refused for hair transplant were included in this study.

Results:

The protocol was able to achieve a platelet concentration of >300% (therapeutic use). Thinning of hair follicle improved in all patients with increased density in the scalp.

Conclusions:

Within the limits of this study, it can be concluded that this is an effective protocol for PRP preparation and PRP definitely helps in hair rejuvenation and is a useful adjunct with hair transplantation though not a replacement to hair transplant.

Keywords: Platelet count, Platelet-rich plasma, Centrifugation

Introduction

Platelet-rich plasma (PRP) is a platelet concentrate which contains proteins such as fibrin, fibronectin and vitronectin that are capable of enhancing cell adhesion and act like a matrix for the formation of bone, connective tissue and epithelium[1].

PRP presently is being used for several indications like musculoskeletal disorders, etc. apart from hair and facial rejuvenation. However, there are controversies in the literature regarding the potential benefits of this procedure in long term. The protocols and surgical techniques used in the preparation and administration of the PRP differ widely[2,3]. Platelet concentration is the single most important factor which can greatly influence the different biological effects[4].

Several protocols for the preparation of PRP have been developed to facilitate its clinical application[5,6,7]. According to Marx[1], PRP should have a platelet concentration 300 to 400% greater than that of the whole blood in order to be considered a "therapeutic PRP." Lower concentrations are reportedly unreliable in enhancing wound healing, while higher concentrations have not been shown to further enhance wound healing[8]. Marx et al[9] stated that a double-centrifugation technique is necessary to truly concentrate platelets from autologous blood. On the other hand, Anitua[5] described using a single-spin technique, although the platelet concentrations obtained by this procedure were not reported. In spite of the amount of platelets, Anitua has demonstrated enhancement and acceleration of bone regeneration and more rapid and predictable soft tissue healing in future sites for implants that were treated with PRP prepared according to a single-spin technique[5]. Other authors have reported obtaining platelet concentrations of 356% using the single-spin technique[10].

Materials and Methods

The experimental protocol was approved by the Ethical committee of Kamal Hospital, Kaushambi, U.P. All the patients who had diffuse thinning of hairs, hair fall or refused for hair transplant were included in this study. All patients were healthy adults with no co-morbities.

PRP preparation

20 ml of blood was taken from each patient. Platelet count was estimated in sample using both automatic cell counter and cross- checked manually

too. Thereafter single centrifugation technique was done at 3000 rpm for 20 minutes. Different layers of the solution containing platelet poor plasma, buffy coat containing rich platelet concentration (PRP) and RBC's were seen as shown in figure 1. Thereafter the PRP was separated from all of them in different tubes. In all the tubes calcium chloride was added 0.05ml/ml of PRP. Thereafter both quantitative and qualitative analysis of platelets was done in PRP samples obtained. Quantitative analysis was again done by using both automatic cell counter and cross checked manually also. Qualitative analysis was also done by preparing smears from the samples.

Platelet study

Quantitative analysis

The platelets in the whole blood and PRP samples was done using automatic cell counter and manually also for cross checking. Platelet concentration was calculated by dividing the platelet count of PRP by the Platelet count of whole blood multiplied by 100.

Qualitative analysis

Smears were prepared using the PRP from all the vials and morphology of platelets was assessed.

Treatment protocol

PRP was used within 30 minutes of its preparation. It was injected in the scalp after local anaesthesia application in the subfollicular plane. Patients were sent home once the PRP session was over and they were in stable condition after checking all the vitals. They were called for review after 4 weeks for next session and told to review earlier if any need arises.

Results

All the data was subjected to statistical analysis and $p<0.05$ was considered significant. All the data was analysed using t-test. P value was significant and the platelet concentration achieved in PRP samples was 310 percent more than the platelet count in whole blood sample as shown in table 1.

Qualitative analysis was done by smear preparation and examination revealed good morphology with minimum acellular debris and aggregates.

The patients were followed up every month for 6 months. All the patients reported improvement in hair fall, thickness of hair and density in areas treated with PRP as can be seen in fig 2 (a,b) and fig 3 (a,b).

Discussion

Different PRP preparation protocols may result in varying platelet concentrations, and thus different biologic effects may occur[8]. The platelet count is the key which decides the regenerative capacity of PRP[11]. In addition, qualitative alterations in the platelets may also affect the regenerative potential of PRP[12]. According to Marx[1], platelets damaged or rendered nonviable by the protocol used to process the PRP will not secrete bioactive growth factors. Thus, the resulting outcome may be disappointing.

Therefore, a "therapeutic PRP" is one that has an average percentage increase of approximately 300-400% in the platelet count[1].

Quantitative assessment was done both manually and by using automatic cell counter as various studies have raised doubts about the level of agreement between manual and automated platelet counts[13-17].

Qualitative analysis of smears is used to evaluate various parameters that are indicative of platelet function, such as changes in morphology, size, shape, staining characteristics, degree of activation and clump formation, distribution of granules and appearance of vacuoles[18]. In the present study, both the platelet concentration in the PRP sample and the final outcome was assessed for best results.

Conclusion

Success of PRP lies primarily in its preparation and the reagents used for the same. Proper selection of technique is essential to yield the best platelet count and morphology.

This conclusion has a **special relevance to aesthetic surgery** since the higher the platelet concentration in PRP used for hair rejuvenation, better the results since growth potential is directly related to platelet concentration which releases active growth factors responsible for growth.

References

1. Marx RE. Platelet-rich plasma: evidence to support its use. J Oral Maxillofac Surg 2004;62:489-496.

2. Weibrich G, Kleis WK, Hitzler WE, Hafner G. Comparison of the platelet concentrate collection system with the plasma rich in growth factors kit to produce platelet-rich plasma: a technical report. Int J Oral Maxillofac Implants 2005;20:118–123.

3. Sánchez AR, Sheridan PJ, Kupp LI. Is platelet-rich plasma the perfect enhancement factor? A current review. Int J Oral Maxillofac Implants 2003;18:93–103.

4. Anitua E, Sánchez M, Nurden AT, Nurden P, Orive G, Andía I. New insights into and novel applications for platelet-rich fibrin therapies. Trends Biotechnol 2006;24:227-234.

5. Anitua E. Plasma rich in growth factors: preliminary results of use in the preparation of sites for implants. Int J Oral Maxillofac Implants 1999;14:529-535.

6. Landesberg R, Roy M, Glickman RS. Quantification of growth factor levels using a simplified method of platelet-rich plasma gel preparation. J Oral Maxillofac Surg 2000;58:297-300.

7. Sonnleitner D, Huemer P, Sullivan DY. A simplified technique for

producing Platelet-rich plasma and Platelet Concentrate for intraoral bone grafting techniques: A technical note. Int J Oral Maxillofac Implants 2000;15:879-882.

8. Tamimi FM, Montalvo S, Tresguerres I, Blanco Jerez L. A comparative study of 2 methods for obtaining platelet-rich plasma. J Oral Maxillofac Surg 2007;65:1084-1093.

9. Marx RE, Carlson ER, Eichstaedt RM, Schimmele SR, Strauss JE, Georgeff KR. Platelet-rich plasma: Growth factor enhancement for bone grafts. Oral Surg Oral Med Oral Pathol Oral Radiol 1998;85:638-646.

10. Eby EW. Platelet-rich plasma: Harvesting with a singlespin centrifuge. J Oral Implantol 2002;28:297-301.

11. Grageda E. Platelet-rich plasma and bone graft materials: a review and a standardized research protocol. Implant Dent. 2004;13:301–309.

12. Messora MR, Nagata MJH, Mariano RC, Dornelles RC, Bomfim SR, Fucini SE, et al. Bone healing in critical-size defects treated with platelet-rich plasma. A histologic and histometric study in rat calvaria. J Periodontal Res. 2008;43:217–223.

13. Hatakeyama M, Beletti ME, Zanetta-Barbosa D, Dechichi P. Radiographic and histomorphometric analysis of bone healing using autogenous graft associated with platelet-rich plasma obtained by 2 different methods. Oral Surg Oral Med Oral Pathol Oral Radiol Endod. 2008;105:e13–e18.

14. Kunz D. Possibilities and limitations of automated platelet counting procedures in the thrombocytopenic range. Semin Thromb Hemost. 2001;27:229–235.

15. Langianni U, Limberti A, Bottari G, Ignesti C, Innocenti V. Evaluation of interferences in electronic platelet count. Quad Sclavo Diagn. 1988;24:197–202.

16. Penev M, Kamenov V, Donkova O, Petkova D. Automatic and manual methods for counting the thrombocytes in the blood. Vutr Boles. 1987;26:109–112.

17. Sutor AH, Grohmann A, Kaufmehl K, Wundisch T. Problems with platelet counting in thrombocytopenia. A rapid manual method to measure low platelet counts. Semin Thromb Hemost. 2001;27:237–243.

18. Halmay D, Sótonyi P, Vajdovich P, Gaál T. Morphological evaluation of canine platelets on Giemsa- and PAS-stained blood smears. Acta Vet Hung. 2005;53:337–350.

Table 1: - Quantitative estimation of platelet count in lakhs(L) both at time of collection (PRE) and after preparation of PRP (PRP sample)

S.No. (Pt.)	Quantitative estimation
A	PRE-1.65L , PRP- 5.20L
B	PRE-1.75 L , PRP- 5.45L
C	PRE- 1.75 L , PRP-5.34L
D	PRE- 1.82 L , PRP-5.51L
E	PRE- 1.85 L , PRP-5.48L
F	PRE- 2.00 L , PRP-5.87L
G	PRE- 1.87 L , PRP-5.82L
H	PRE- 1.65 L , PRP-5.13L
I	PRE- 1.80L , PRP-5.33 L
J	PRE- 1.56 L , PRP-5.21 L
K	PRE- 1.77 L , PRP-5.42 L
L	PRE- 2.00 L , PRP-5.58 L
M	PRE- 1.70 L , PRP-5.52L
N	PRE- 1.65 L , PRP-5.65 L
O	PRE- 1.85 L , PRP-5.91 L
P	PRE-1.91 L , PRP-5.82 L
Q	PRE- 1.65 L , PRP-5.18 L
R	PRE- 2.08 L , PRP-5.57 L
S	PRE- 1.60 L , PRP-5.43 L
T	PRE- 1.75 L , PRP-5.79 L
TOTAL	PRE- 35.7L , PRP- 110.2L
PLATELET - PRP/PRE X 100	310%
CONCENTRATION	

Figure 1: - showing the 3 different layers of the solution

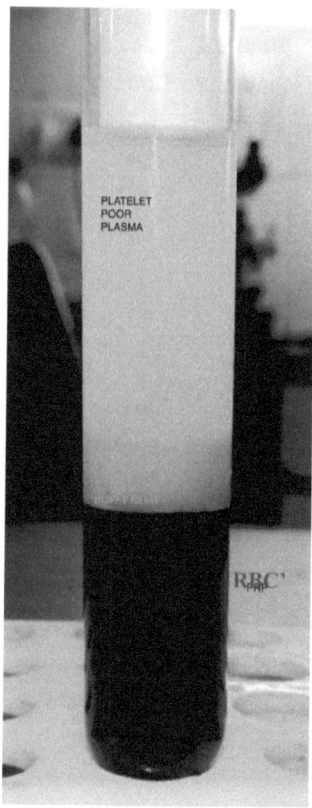

Figure 2: - Pre and post PRP image showing increased follicular density, thickness and length covering the previous bald scalp.

PRE-PRP

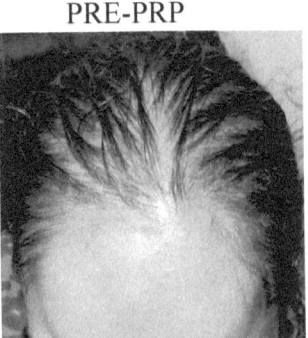

POST PRP

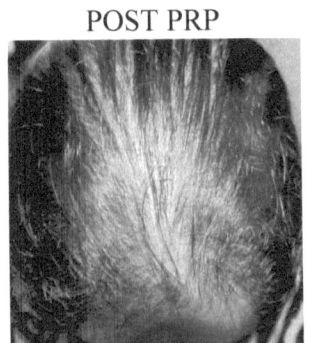

Fig 3: - Pre and post PRP image showing increased follicular density per sq cm.

PRE-PRP POST PRP

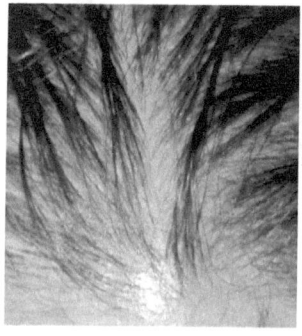
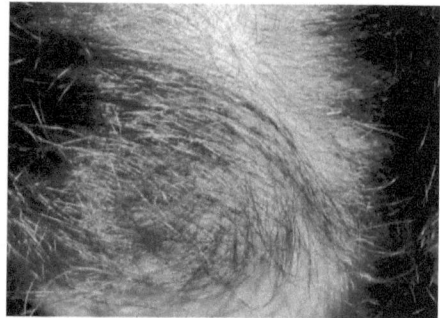

PRP in Chronic Alopecia Areata-Our Centre Experience

Abstract

Alopecia areata is a common, nonscarring, autoimmune disease that can affect any hair- bearing area. Its pathogenesis is not well defined and it can present as a single patch or multiple patches or sometimes so extensive and result in alopecia totalis and universalis. Various treatment options have been available for this disease but none of them are curative and all have some or the other side effects associated with long-term use. This article illustrates a definitive role of PRP in treating chronic alopecia areata infection.

Keywords

Alopecia Areata (AA)

PRP- Platelet Rich Plasma

Introduction

Alopecia areata is a common, nonscarring, autoimmune disease that can affect any hair-bearing area. Though various line of managements have been described for this infection [1-24], all have significant relapse rate with side effects too. In this report we wish to discuss about 20 patients of chronic alopecia aereata infection, biopsy proven, who had already taken 2 years of various therapies with almost no results.

Platelet rich plasma (PRP) is an autologous preparation of platelets in concentrated plasma. It has been investigated in several disciplines of medicine for its role in wound healing. In our centre we have treated about 20 patients of alopecia aereata with PRP alone without any side effects and with good results as seen in figure 1 (a,b).

We decided to use platelet rich plasma (PRP) for improvement of the patient's outcome as we had success in the use of PRP for hair rejuvenation and cicatricial alopecia [25,26]. There has been only one double-blinded, placebo and active-controlled, half-head, parallel group study on 45 patients to evaluate the efficacy and safety of PRP in Alopecia Aereata patients [27]. This study concluded that PRP is a safe and alternative treatment for Alopecia Aereata, but further controlled trials are needed to validate the findings.

Materials and Methods

This is a prospective study that was conducted at Kamal hospital, Kaushambi in which all the 20 patients who attended the out patient department were enrolled for the study. All the patients had h/o patches and taken various line of treatments for a duration of 2 years. All the patients were biopsy proven positive for alopecia aereata infection. There was no specific randomization done since all of them were healthy young adults. All the patients age ranged from 25-35 years and none of them had any co-morbities. All the patients were explained about the procedure in detail. Consent form was signed by each patient. All the patients were followed up at 4 weekly intervals for a duration 0f 6 months and then at the end of one year. All the patients received 6 sessions of PRP. Ethical committee approval was taken prior to the commencement of the study.

Treatment protocol

25 ml of blood was taken from each patient and the PRP solution obtained from the lab was used within 30 minutes of its preparation. It was injected in the scalp after local anaesthesia application in the

subfollicular plane. Patients were sent home once the PRP session was over and they were in stable condition after checking all the vitals. They were called for review after 4 weeks for next session and told to review earlier if any need arises. All the patients received 6 sessions of PRP at 4 weekly intervals. Patients were reviewed every month for 6 months and then at the end of one year.

Results

Out of 20 patients, one patient had a relapse and his hair regrowth was also minimum [fig.2 a, b, c]. None of the patients had any side effects and all of them tolerated the procedure well.

Discussion

Proper counseling of the patient is very important before starting treatment for this disease, since it is associated with recurrences very commonly. All the treatments available as of today are associated with both relapses and side effects, which affects the psychosocial life of the patients in long run.

Various treatments are available for alopecia aereata infection. The effect of a single intralesional corticosteroid injection has been observed to persist for up to 9 months in few studies[2], reported relapse rates were 29% in limited alopecia areata and 72% in alopecia totalis during a 3-month follow-up period[1]. The reported relapse rate of topical steroids is 37%–63%[4,5]. In a placebo-controlled, double-blind study, hair regrowth was observed in 63.6% and 35.7% of the minoxidil-treated and placebo groups, respectively[6]. In another study, hair regrowth was achieved in 38% and 81% of patients treated with 1% and 5% topical minoxidil, respectively[7]. Side effects include contact dermatitis and facial hypertrichosis. Various forms of systemic corticosteroids have been used in different regimens. In one study, a once-monthly oral pulse of 300 mg prednisone induced a complete response in 41% of patients [19]. A similar effect has been reported in a placebo-controlled trial of oral prednisolone 200 mg once weekly in the treatment of extensive alopecia areata [20]. The relapse rate was 25%, and side effects of the therapy were noted in 55% of patients [20]. Other medications include Methotrexate with relapse rate of more than 50%; Cyclosporine with a high relapse rate of almost 100% [24]; Azathioprine and others.

In contrast our study showed relapse in just one case and no side effects in any of the 20 treated patients. Though we have achieved initial success with PRP, still more follow up is required and more studies needed to validate the final results.

Conclusion

We wish to conclude that PRP has a definite role in treating alopecia aereata infections. But still more long term follow up and studies are required for further validation of results and labeling it as a 100 percent cure for people suffering from alopecia aereata with recurrences which are so common.

References

1. Abell E, Munro DD. Intralesional treatment of alopecia areata with triamcinolone acetonide by jet injector. Br J Dermatol. 1973;88(1):55–59.

2. Orentreich N, Sturm HM, Weidman AI, Pelzig A. Local injection of steroids and hair regrowth in alopecias. Arch Dermatol. 1960;82:894–902.

3. Mancuso G, Balducci A, Casadio C, et al. Efficacy of betamethasone valerate foam formulation in comparison with betamethasone dipropionate lotion in the treatment of mild-to-moderate alopecia areata: a multicenter, prospective, randomized, controlled, investigator-blinded trial. Int J Dermatol. 2003;42(7):572–575.

4. Tosti A, Piraccini BM, Pazzaglia M, Vincenzi C. Clobetasol propionate 0.05% under occlusion in the treatment of alopecia totalis/universalis. J Am Acad Dermatol. 2003;49(1):96–98.

5. Pascher F, Kurtin S, Andrade R. Assay of 0.2 percent fluocinolone acetonide cream for alopecia areata and totalis. Efficacy and side effects including histologic study of the ensuing localized acneform response. Dermatologica. 1970;141(3):193–202.

6. Price VH. Double-blind, placebo-controlled evaluation of topical minoxidil in extensive alopecia areata. J Am Acad Dermatol. 1987;16(3 Pt 2):730–736.

7. Fiedler-Weiss VC. Topical minoxidil solution (1% and 5%) in the treatment of alopecia areata. J Am Acad Dermatol. 1987;16(3 Pt 2):745–748.

8. Fiedler-Weiss VC, Buys CM. Evaluation of anthralin in the treatment of alopecia areata. Arch Dermatol. 1987;123(11):1491–1493.

9. Fiedler VC, Wendrow A, Szpunar GJ, Metzler C, DeVillez RL. Treatment-resistant alopecia areata. Response to combination therapy with minoxidil plus anthralin. Arch Dermatol. 1990;126(6):756–759.

10. Aghaei S. Topical immunotherapy of severe alopecia areata with diphenylcyclopropenone (DPCP): experience in an Iranian population. BMC Dermatol. 2005;5:6.

11. Francomano M, Seidenari S. Urticaria after topical immunotherapy with diphenylcyclopropenone. Contact Dermatitis. 2002;47(5):310–311.

12. Coronel-Perez IM, Rodriguez-Rey EM, Camacho-Martinez FM. Latanoprost in the treatment of eyelash alopecia in alopecia areata universalis. J Eur Acad Dermatol Venereol. 2010;24(4):481–485.

13. Rashidi T, Mahd AA. Treatment of persistent alopecia areata with sulfasalazine. Int J Dermatol. 2008;47(8):850–852.

14. Aghaei S. An uncontrolled, open label study of sulfasalazine in severe alopecia areata. Indian J Dermatol Venereol Leprol. 2008;74(6):611–613.

15. Ellis CN, Brown MF, Voorhees JJ. Sulfasalazine for alopecia areata. J Am Acad Dermatol. 2002;46(4):541–544.

16. Taylor CR, Hawk JL. PUVA treatment of alopecia areata partialis, totalis and universalis: audit of 10 years' experience at St John's Institute of Dermatology. Br J Dermatol. 1995;133(6):914–918.

17. Mohamed Z, Bhouri A, Jallouli A, Fazaa B, Kamoun MR, Mokhtar I. Alopecia areata treatment with a phototoxic dose of UVA and topical 8-methoxypsoralen. J Eur Acad Dermatol Venereol. 2005;19(5):552–555.

18. Broniarczyk-Dyla G, Wawrzycka-Kaflik A, Dubla-Berner M, Prusinska- Bratos M. Effects of psoralen-UV-A-Turban in alopecia areata. Skinmed. 2006;5(2):64–68.

19. Ait Ourhroui M, Hassam B, Khoudri I. Treatment of alopecia areata with prednisone in a once-monthly oral pulse. Ann Dermatol Venereol. 2010;137(8–9):514–518. French.

20. Kar BR, Handa S, Dogra S, Kumar B. Placebo-controlled oral pulse prednisolone therapy in alopecia areata. J Am Acad Dermatol. 2005;52(2):287–290.

21. Kurosawa M, Nakagawa S, Mizuashi M, et al. A comparison of the efficacy, relapse rate and side effects among three modalities of systemic corticosteroid therapy for alopecia areata. Dermatology. 2006;212(4):361–365.

22. Sharma VK, Gupta S. Twice weekly 5 mg dexamethasone oral pulse in the treatment of extensive alopecia areata. J Dermatol. 1999;26(9):562–565.

23. Luggen P, Hunziker T. High-dose intravenous corticosteroid pulse therapy in alopecia areata: own experience compared with the literature. J Dtsch Dermatol Ges. 2008;6(5):375–378. German.

24. Gupta AK, Ellis CN, Cooper KD, et al. Oral cyclosporine for the treatment of alopecia areata. A clinical and immunohistochemical analysis. J Am Acad Dermatol. 1990;22(2 Pt 1):242–250.

25. **Singh S**. Platelet Rich Plasma- Protocol for its preparation and its role in hair rejuvenation. The Aestheticians Journal, Oct 2013. Vol 3, Issue 10: 40-42.

26) **Singh S**. Role of Platelet Rich Plasma in Primary Cicatricial alopecia. The Aestheticians Journal Feb 2014, Vol 4, Issue 1: 42-44.

27) Trink A1, Sorbellini E, Bezzola P, Rodella L, Rezzani R, Ramot Y, Rinaldi F. A randomized, double blind, placebo- and active-controlled, half-head study to evaluate the effects of platelet-rich plasma on alopecia areata. Br J Dermatol. 2013 Sep; 169(3): 690-4.

Figure 1a: - Showing Pre-intervention state of the patient with alopecia areata

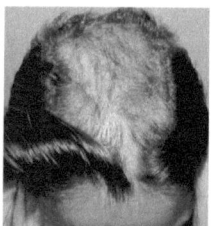

Figure 1b: - Showing Post-PRP status- note the improved sustained hair growth at the end of 1 year

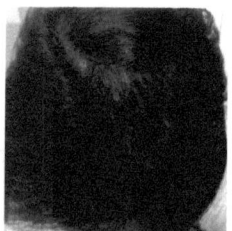

Figure 2a: - Showing Pre-intervention state of the patient with alopecia areata

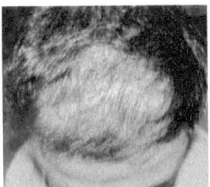

Figure 2b: - Showing Post-PRP status- note the improved hair growth at the end of 6 months.

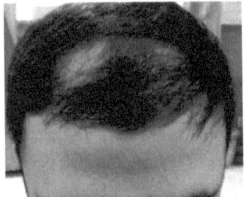

Figure 2c: - Showing Post-PRP status- note the relapse at the end of 1 year.

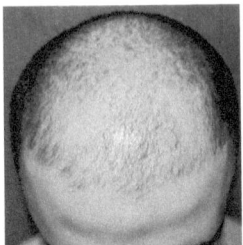

Role of PRP in Primary Cicatricial Alopecia

Abstract

Alopecia in the scalp region leads to low self-esteem and psychosocial embarrassment for an individual. Hence an early diagnosis to the cause of alopecia must be established and an aggressive treatment protocol are crucial in the management of scarring alopecia. This article presents the treatment options in cicatricial alopecia and the role of Platelet Rich Plasma (PRP) in the same.

Keywords: Cicatricial alopecia, primary cicatricial alopecia, secondary cicatricial alopecia, stable alopecia, unstable alopecia, Platelet rich plasma (PRP).

Introduction

Cicatricial alopecias (CAs) or scarring alopecias are a group of uncommon inflammatory hair loss disorders, which are characterized by permanent destruction of hair follicles. Clinically there is loss of visible follicular ostia in the scarring area, with or without epidermal atrophy and histologically there is absence of pilosebaceous structures which are replaced by fibrous tracts[1-5].

Classification

The causes of CA are broadly classified as primary, secondary, and hereditary or developmental defects[4-6]. In PCA, there is irreversible hair loss from the affected site on scalp and the inflammatory cells targets and destroys the stem cells in the bulge area of hair follicles[4]. In SCA, the hair follicles are secondarily damaged as a result of more generalized destructive process within the skin[5]. The causes of SCA are trauma (burns, radiation, traction), any infiltrative processes (morphoea, scleroderma, sarcoidosis, neoplasias), and infections (bacterial, fungal, viral, mycobacterial)[6].

Another classification categorises CA into "stable" and "unstable" type[8]. "Stable" CAs are secondary to isolated events that cause permanent scarring in a hair-bearing region. Whereas "unstable" cicatricial alopecias (UCAs) are secondary to disorders that have a tendency to progress and recur intermittently over the course of time.

Pathogenesis

The pathogenesis of PCA revolves mainly around the destruction of slow-cycling, pluripotent hair follicle stem cells (HFSCs)[9]. These HFSCs are located in the 'bulge' region of hair follicle in outer root sheath (i.e., at the site of attachment of the arrector pili muscle to the outer root sheath). The newer insights into the pathogenesis of PCA mainly involves the HFSCs destruction theories, impairment of self maintenance of HFSCs, alteration of lipid metabolism, neurogenic inflammation theory, environment and genetic factors[4, 11-30].

Clinical features

In this condition, the patient presents with an unusual clinical pattern of alopecia with severe loss of hairs, most commonly involving the occipital scalp (40% cases), other being temporal area. On close examination of scalp, there is no clinical appreciable scarring, atrophy, or erythema.

Diagnosis

One of the mainstay in diagnosis and management of cicatricial alopecia is histopathological examination. Histopathology of scalp is an essential tool in distinguishing CA from non-CA and in diagnosing the different PCA depending upon the inflammatory infiltrate. Multiple biopsy samples are obtained from active sites and carefully sectioned both vertically and transversely[2]. Transverse sections enable both qualitative (e.g., inflammatory change, fibrosis) and quantitative (e.g., hair follicle numbers, size, phase of hair cycle) examination of scalp biopsy samples[31].

Based upon the histopathological picture, the CAs are divided mainly into lymphocyte-mediated primary cicatricial alopecia (LMPCA), neutrophil-mediated primary cicatricial alopecia (NMPCA), and mixed CA[7].

Management

PCA provides both the diagnostic and therapeutic dilemma to the treating surgeon. The aim of treatment currently focuses the reduction of symptoms and to reduce or stop the progression of the disease. A general rule followed is to treat LMPCA with immunosuppression and NMPCA with antimicrobials or dapsone[32]. We have been using exclusively PRP for primary cicatricial alopecia cases.

Surgical treatment of scarring alopecia includes hair transplantation, scalp reduction surgeries, tissue expansion and flap surgeries[8]. Decision for surgical treatment is based upon the stability of the CA, because best results can only be obtained in stable cicatricial alopecia cases[8]. The other factors that require consideration before planning the surgical treatment for CA includes vigilance regarding possible evolution of future androgenetic alopecia in the patient under treatment, availability of donor hairs and donor-recipient area ratio, vascular supply to the recipient area, scalp laxity, patient's healing characteristics, and location of the subsequent scars[8].

Recent innovation has been the use of Platelet rich plasma (PRP) therapy for hair rejuvenation. We are using PRP for primary cicatricial alopecia, both unstable and stable cases. We have seen great improvement in the scalp texture and hair regrowth as evident from figure 1a and 1b. Even in unstable cases, PRP helps to achieve stability. For residual cases, which have attained stability for a period of 2 years, hair transplant can be used as a definitive option.

Conclusion

PRP is a definitive treatment option for cases of PCA and should be used in addition to the previous protocols for PCA. Secondly stability of minimum 2 years is a must to achieve definitive cure in form of hair transplant. But still a great deal of research is required in this field for the final cure.

References

1. Whiting DA. Cicatricial alopecia: Clinico-pathological findings and treatment. Clin Dermatol 2001;19:211-5.
2. Tan E, Martinka M, Ball N, Shapiro J. Primary cicatricial alopecias: Clinicopathology of 112 cases. J Am Acad Dermatol 2004;50:25-32.
3. Griffin LL, Michaelides C, Griffiths CE, Paus R, Harries MJ. Primary cicatricial alopecias: A UK survey. Br J Dermatol 2012;167:692-705.
4. Ohyama M. Primary cicatricial alopecia: Recent advances in understanding and management. J Dermatol 2012;39:18-26.
5. Paus R, Olsen E, Messenger A. Hair growth disorders. In: Wolff K, Goldsmith LA, Katz SI, Gilchrest BA, Paller AS, Leffell DJ, editors. Fitzpatrick's Dermatology in General Medicine. 7th ed. New York: McGraw-Hill; 2008. p. 753.
6. Sinclair RD. Acquired cicatricial alopecia. In: Burns T, Breathnach SM, Cox N, Griffiths CE, editors. Rook's Textbook of Dermatology. 8th ed. Oxford: Wiley-Blackwill Publishing; 2010. p. 66.38-66.52.
7. Olsen EA, Bergfeld WF, Cotsarelis G, Price VH, Shapiro J, Sinclair R, et al.

Summary of North American Hair Research Society (NAHRS)-sponsored Workshop on Cicatricial Alopecia, Duke University Medical Center, February 10 and 11, 2001. J Am Acad Dermatol 2003;48:103-10.

8. Unger W, Unger R, Wesley C. The surgical treatment of cicatricial alopecia. Dermatol Ther 2008;21:295-311.

9. Sellheyer K, Bergfeld WF. Histopathologic evaluation of alopecias. Am J Dermatopathol 2006;28:236-59.

10. Lavker RM, Sun TT, Oshima H, Barrandon Y, Akiyama M, Ferraris C, et al. Hair follicle stem cells. J Invest Dermatol 2003;8:28-38.

11. Harries MJ, Paus R. The pathogenesis of primary cicatricial alopecias. Am J Pathol 2010;177:2152-62.

12. Cotsarelis G. Epithelial stem cells: A folliculocentric view. J Invest Dermatol 2006;126:1459-68.

13. Paus R, Cotsarelis G. The biology of hair follicles. N Engl J Med. 1999;341:491-7.

14. Pozdnyakova O, Mahalingam M. Involvement of the bulge region in primary scarring alopecia. J Cutan Pathol 2008;35:922-5.

15. Al-Refu K, Edward S, Ingham E, Goodfield M. Expression of hair follicle stem cells detected by cytokeratin 15 stain: Implications for pathogenesis of the scarring process in cutaneous lupus erythematosus. Br J Dermatol 2009;160:1188-96.

16. Cotsarelis G, Millar SE. Towards a molecular understanding of hair loss

and its treatment. Trends Mol Med 2001;7:293-301.

17. McElwee KJ. Etiology of cicatricial alopecias: A basic science point of view. Dermatol Ther 2008;21:212-20.
18. Nijhof JG, Braun KM, Giangreco A. The cell-surface marker MTS24 identifies a novel population of follicular keratinocytes with characteristics of progenitor cells. Development 2006; 133:3027-37.
19. Jensen KB, Collins CA, Nascimento E. Lrig1 expression defines a distinct multipotent stem cell population in mammalian epidermis. Cell Stem Cell 2009;4:427-39.
20. Amoh Y, Li L, Katsuoka K, Penman S, Hoffman RM. Multipotent nestin-positive, keratin-negative hair-follicle bulge stem cells can form neurons. Proc Natl Acad Sci USA 2005;102:5530-4.
21. Jaks V, Barker N, Kasper M, van Es JH, Snippert HJ, Clevers H, et al. Lgr5 marks cycling, yet long-lived, hair follicle stem cells. Nat Genet 2008;40:1291-9.
22. Snippert HJ, Haegebarth A, Kasper M, Jaks V, van Es JH, Barker N, et al. Lgr6 marks stem cells in the hair follicle that generate all cell lineages of the skin. Science 2010;327:1385-9.
23. Harries MJ, Meyer KC, Chaudhry IH, Griffiths CE, Paus R. Does collapse of immune privilege in the hair-follicle bulge play a role in the pathogenesis of primary cicatricial alopecia? Clin Exp Dermatol 2010;35:637-44.
24. Baima B, Sticherling M. Apoptosis in different cutaneous manifestations of lupus erythematosus. Br J Dermatol 2001;144:958-66.
25. Pablos JL, Santiago B, Galindo M, Carreira PE, Ballestin C, Gomez-Reino JJ. Keratinocyte apoptosis and p53 expression in cutaneous lupus and dermatomyositis. J Pathol 1999;188:63-8.
26. Nakajima M, Nakajima A, Kayagaki N, Honda M, Yagita H, Okumura K. Expression of Fas ligand and its receptor in

cutaneous lupus: implication in tissue injury. Clin Immunol Immunopathol 1997;83:223-9.

27. Zheng Y, Eilertsen KJ, Ge L, Zhang L, Sundberg JP, Prouty SM, *et al.* Scd1 is expressed in sebaceous glands and is disrupted in the asebia mouse. Nat Genet 1999;23:268-70.

28. Sundberg JP, Boggess D, Sundberg BA, Eilertsen K, Parimoo S, Filippi M, *et al.* Asebia-2J (Scd1(ab2J)): a new allele and a model for scarring alopecia. Am J Pathol 2000;156:2067-75.

29. Stenn KS. Insights from the asebia mouse: A molecular sebaceous gland defect leading to cicatricial alopecia. J Cutan Pathol 2001;28:445-7.

30. Karnik P, Tekeste Z, McCormick TS, Gilliam AC, Price VH, Cooper KD, *et al.* Hair follicle stem cell-specific PPARγ deletion causes scarring alopecia. J Invest Dermatol 2009;129:1243-57.

31. Sperling LC. Scarring alopecia and the dermatopathologist. J Cutan Pathol 2001;28:333-42.

32. Harries MJ, Sinclair RD, Donald-Hull M, Whiting DA, Griffiths CE, Paus R. Management of primary cicatricial alopecias: Options for treatment. Br J Dermatol 2008;159:1-22.

Figure 1a

Pre-intervention stage

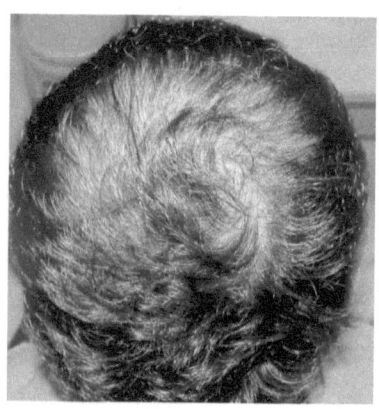

Figure 1b

Post intervention stage with PRP-marked improvement can be appreciated.

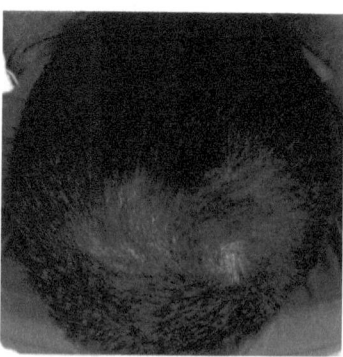

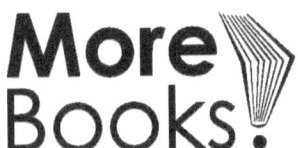
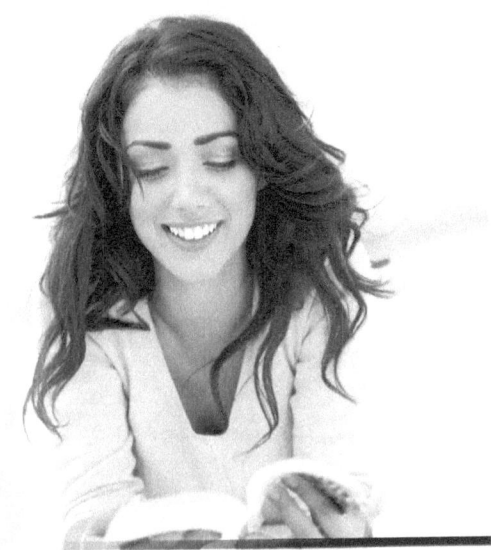

i want morebooks!

Buy your books fast and straightforward online - at one of the world's fastest growing online book stores! Environmentally sound due to Print-on-Demand technologies.

Buy your books online at

www.get-morebooks.com

Kaufen Sie Ihre Bücher schnell und unkompliziert online – auf einer der am schnellsten wachsenden Buchhandelsplattformen weltweit! Dank Print-On-Demand umwelt- und ressourcenschonend produziert.

Bücher schneller online kaufen

www.morebooks.de

OmniScriptum Marketing DEU GmbH
Heinrich-Böcking-Str. 6-8
D - 66121 Saarbrücken
Telefax: +49 681 93 81 567-9

info@omniscriptum.de
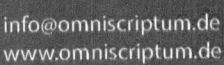
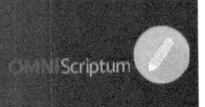

www.ingramcontent.com/pod-product-compliance
Lightning Source LLC
Chambersburg PA
CBHW031552210526

45464CB00003B/1268